Mommy Feeds Baby

Written and Illustrated by Christy Jo Hendricks

Mommy Feeds Baby
Published by 3B Publishing

ISBN-13:978-0-9831848-0-5

Library of Congress Control Number: 2011920157
Printed in USA

This book is available at special quantity discounts for bulk purchases, promotions, gift purposes, fundraisers, and educational use. Special books can also be created to fit specific needs. For information contact 3B Publishing via email at BBBPublishing@msn.com, or visit the website www.birthingandbreastfeeding.com

Because of Derek, Ally and JoJo,

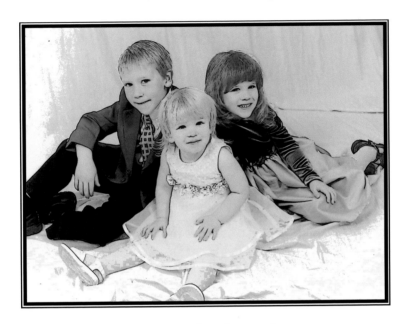

Mommy fed Babies.

Dedicated to my children—Derek, Allyson, and Joanna—for teaching me about the bond created through breastfeeding and for making me a mom—the best position I have ever held; and to my husband, David, who could have written a volume of books: "Daddy...Plays with, Bathes, Cuddles, Protects, Changes, Teaches, Sings to, Rocks...Baby."
You made sure you didn't miss out on a thing.

A very special thanks to all the families who allowed me to photograph their everyday routines as they held, nurtured, and fed their children.

Because Baby wants
to have a snack,

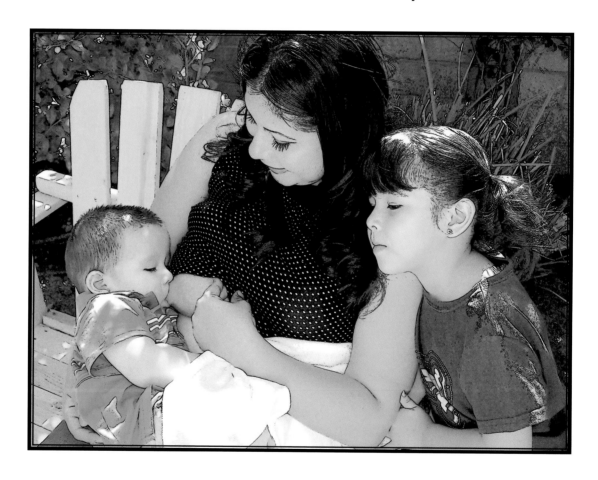

Mommy feeds Baby.

Because Mommy likes to keep Baby close,

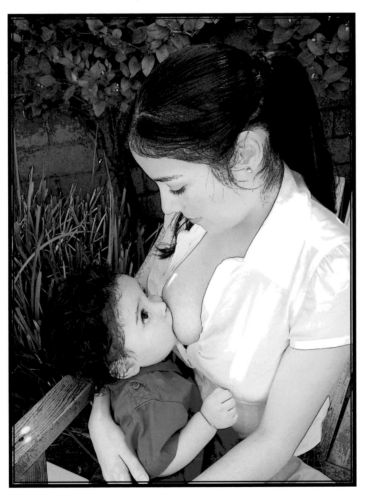

Mommy feeds Baby.

Because Mommy cares
what Baby eats,

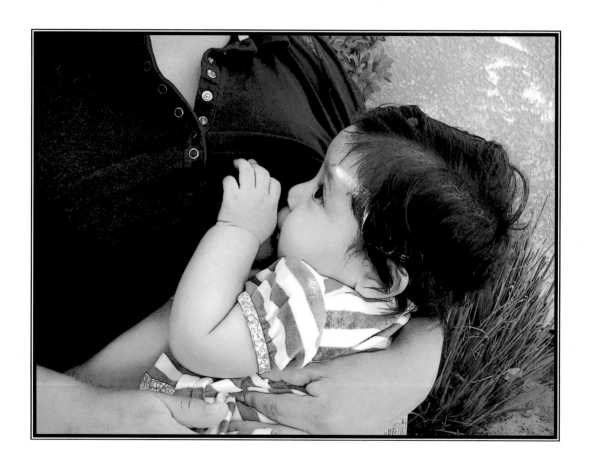

Mommy feeds Baby.

Because Baby gets hungry
when we are out,

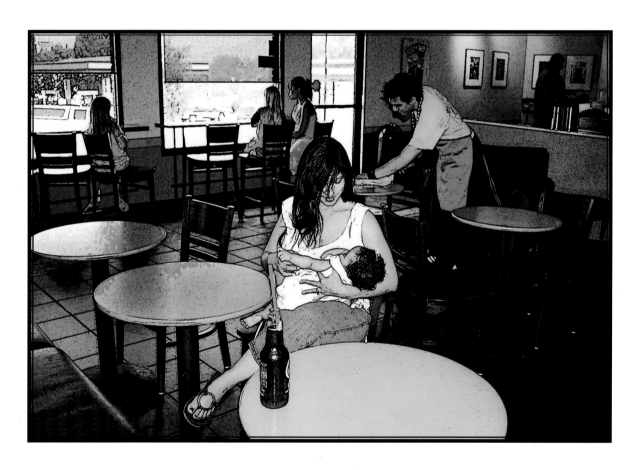

Mommy feeds Baby.

Because touch is
so important to Baby,

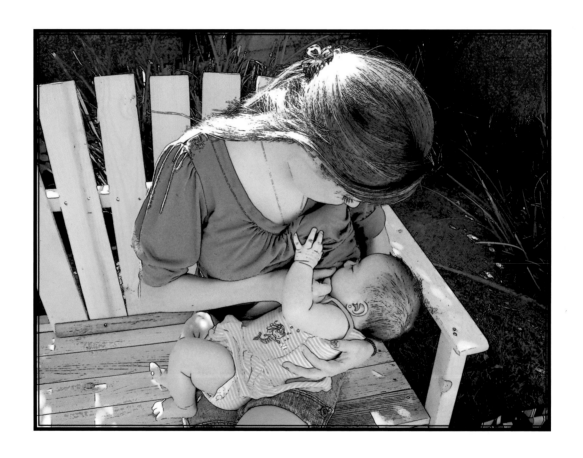

Mommy feeds Baby.

Because Baby is part
of the family,

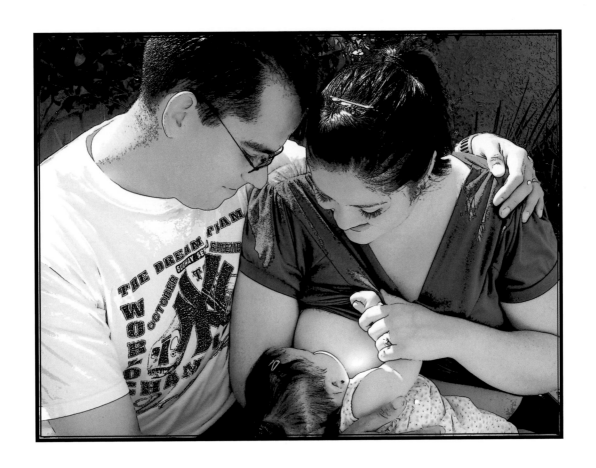

Mommy feeds Baby.

Because Baby needs
to feel safe and cared for,

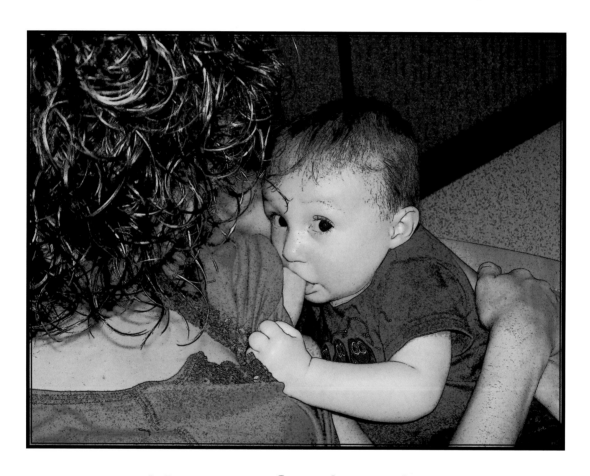

Mommy feeds Baby.

Because Mommy knows
what is best,

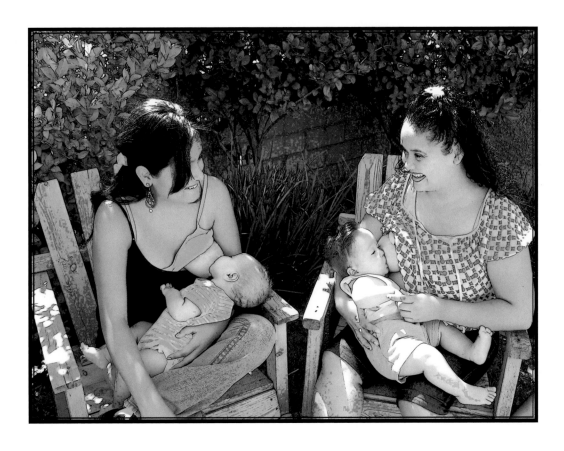

Mommy feeds Baby.

Because I have
a new baby brother,

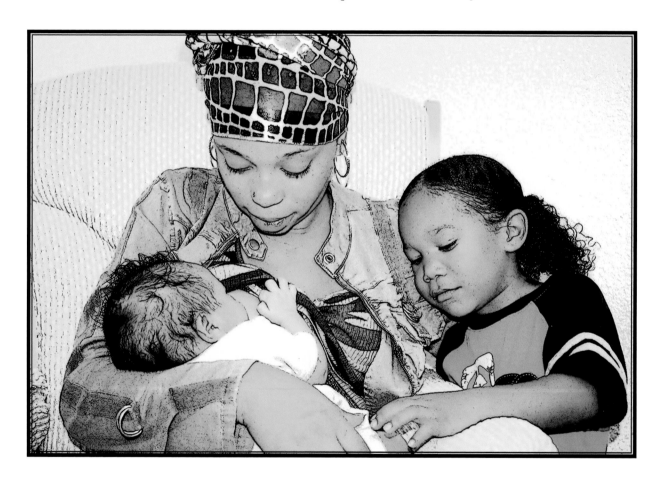

Mommy feeds Baby.

Because Mommy loves Baby,

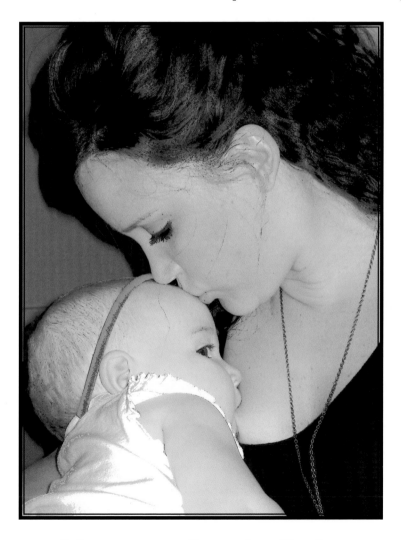

Mommy feeds Baby.

Because Baby will soon
be all grown up,

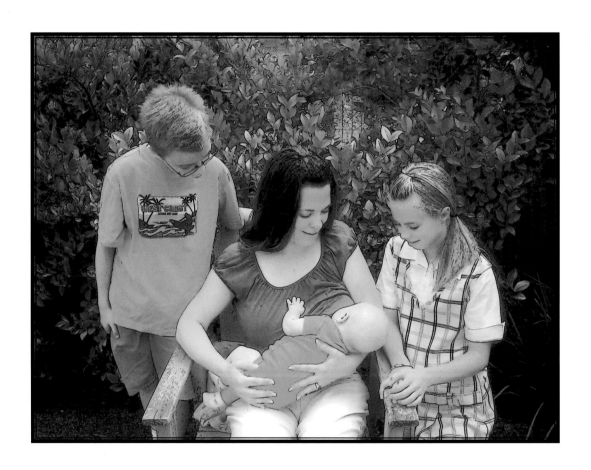

Mommy feeds Baby.

Because Mommy likes
to rest with Baby,

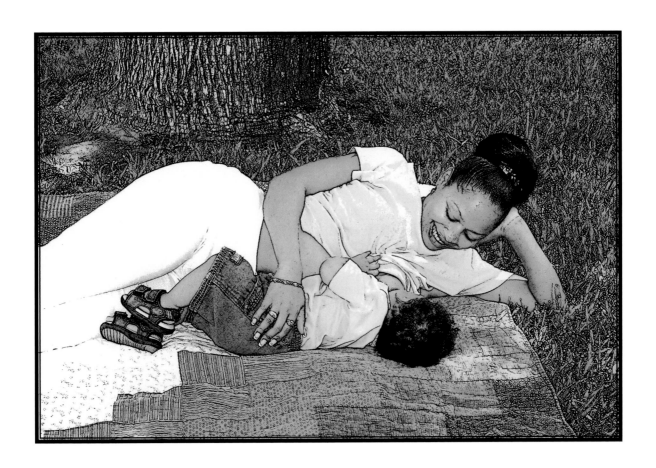

Mommy feeds Baby.

Because Baby is hungry
when he wakes up,

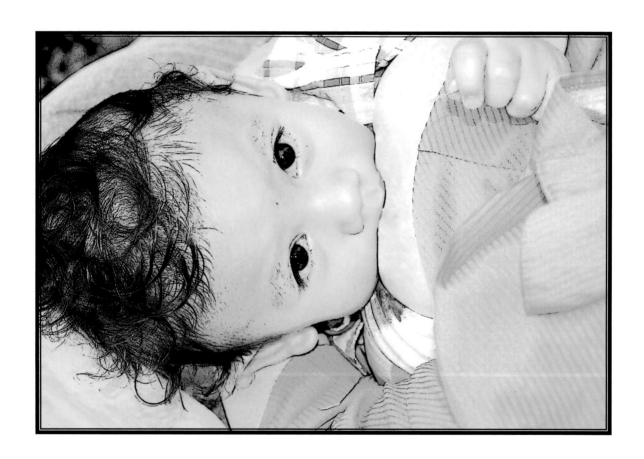

Mommy feeds Baby.

Because Mommy and Baby have a special bond,

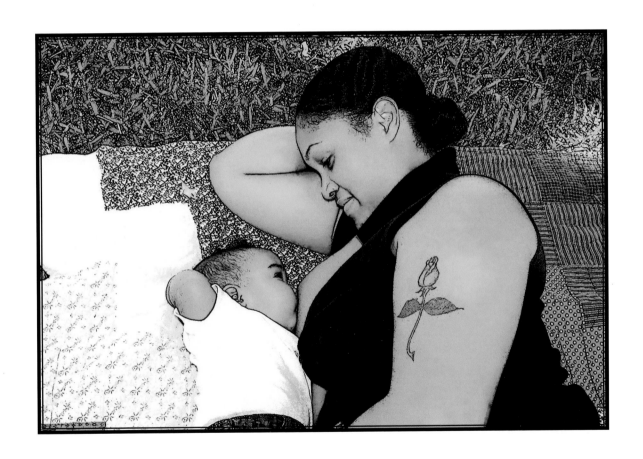

Mommy feeds Baby.

Because Baby looks
up to Mommy,

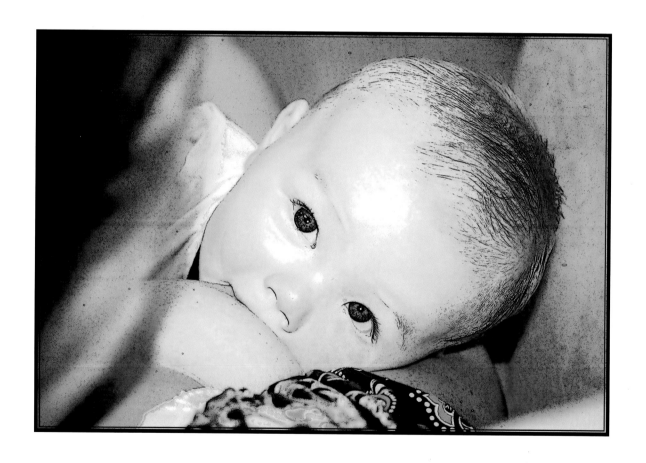

Mommy feeds Baby.

Because Mommy makes sure
we eat healthy food,

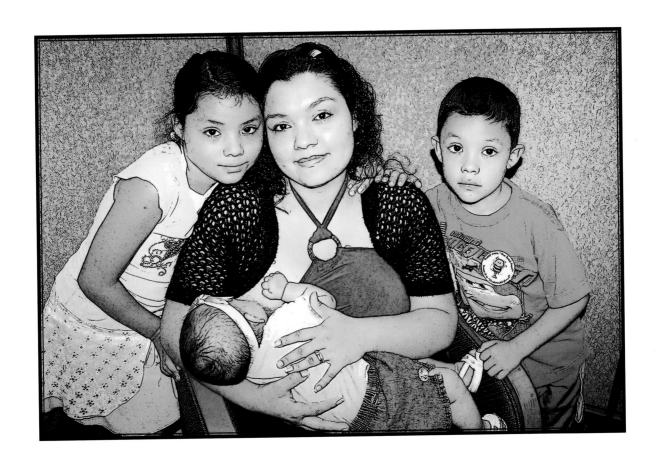

Mommy feeds Baby.

Because Daddy wants
what is best for Baby,

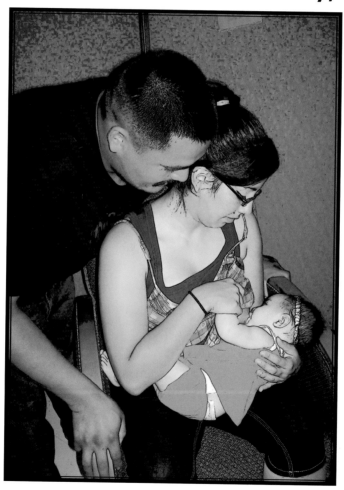

Mommy feeds Baby.

Because Baby likes
to hold Mommy,

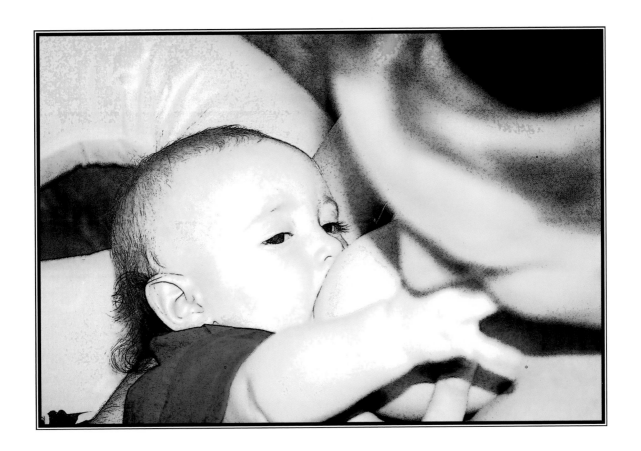

Mommy feeds Baby.

Because doing things
together is fun,

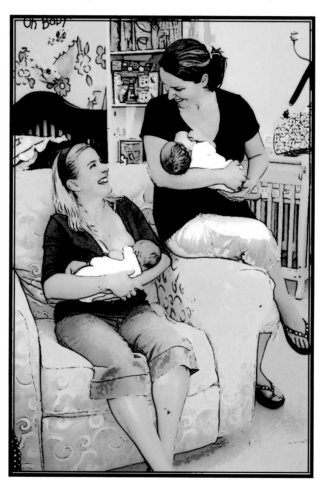

Mommy feeds Baby.

Because Baby is getting
very sleepy,

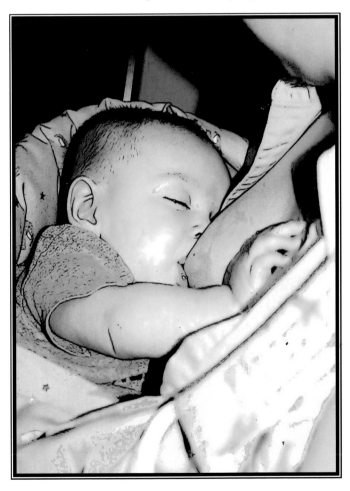

Mommy feeds Baby.

Because Baby belongs
with Mommy,

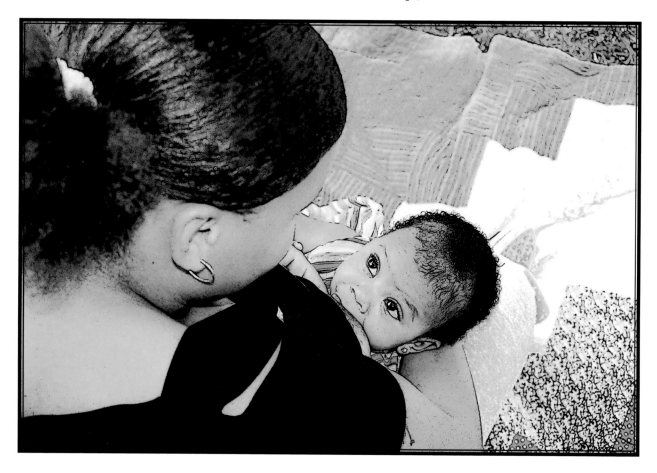

Mommy feeds Baby.

Because Baby is happy
in Mommy's arms,

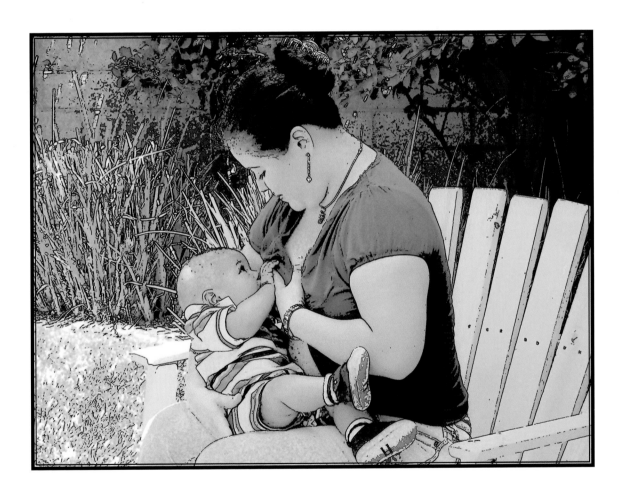

Mommy feeds Baby.

Because Baby is carried in a sling,

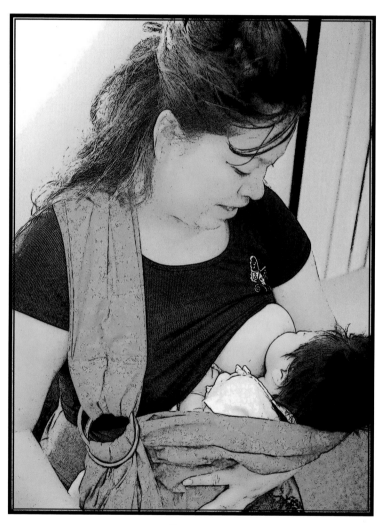

Mommy feeds Baby.

Because Big Sister is watching,

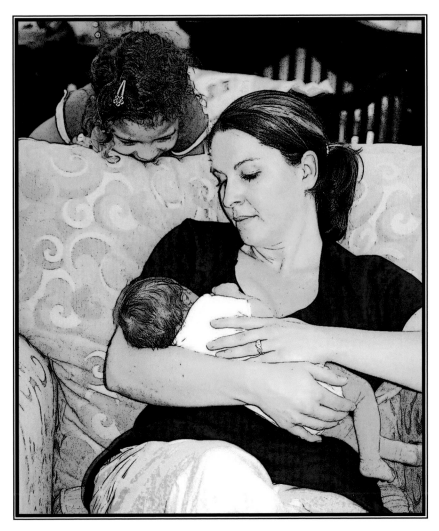

Mommy feeds Baby.

Because it is a nice day
to sit in the park,

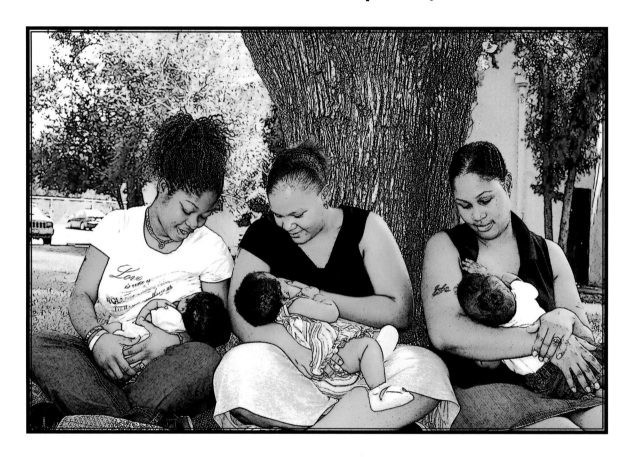

Mommy feeds Baby.

Because Mommy wants
to protect Baby,

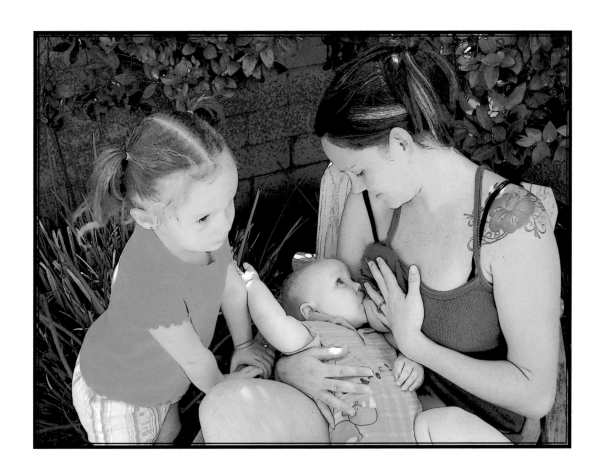

Mommy feeds Baby.

Because being with Mommy
is so much fun,

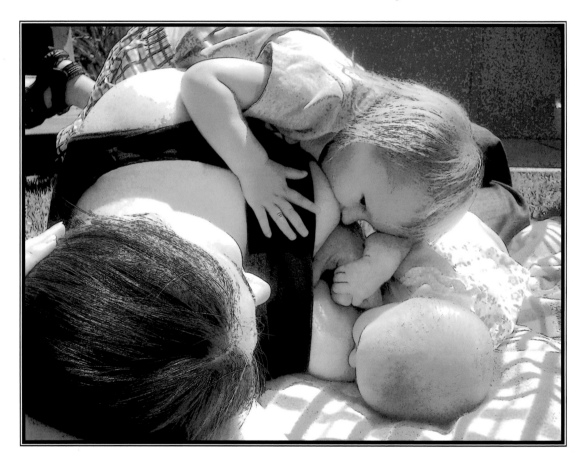

Mommy feeds Baby.

Because mommies everywhere
are caring for babies,

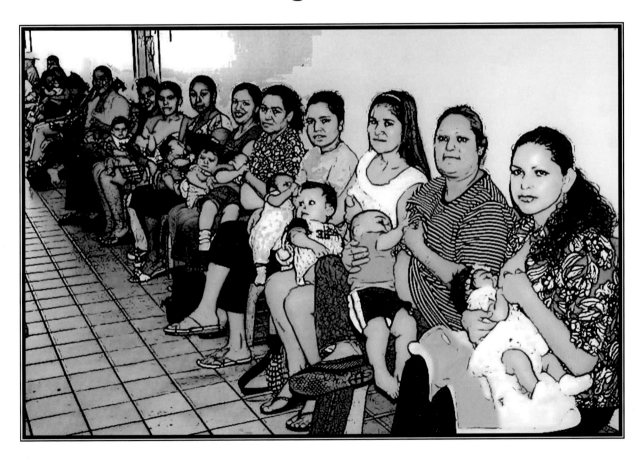

Mommies feed Babies.

Because

---

*Complete the book with your own
"Mommy feeds Baby" photo and verse.*

Mommy feeds Baby.